DINE SMART, WIN BIG.

Burn Fat, Improve your Metabolism and Prolong Your Life.

BONUS:Guided Meditation Scripts for Mindful Eating: Nourishing Your Body And Soul.

BY

Catherine. J. Norris

Copyright © 2024 by Catherine.J.Norris

certain other noncommercial uses permitted by copyright law.

In no event will we be liable for any loss or damage, including without limitation, indirect or consequential loss or damage, or any loss or damage whatsoever arising from loss of data or profits arising out of, or in connection with, the use of this book[Beyond Sweat and Tears].

Through this book [Beyond Sweat and Tears], you may be able to link to other websites that are not under the control of [Catherine.J.Norris]. We have no control over the nature, content, and availability of those sites. The inclusion of any links does not necessarily imply a recommendation or endorse the views expressed within them.

Every effort is made to keep [this book, website, or other content format] up and running smoothly. However, Catherine.J.Norris takes no responsibility for, and will not be liable for, [this book, website, or other content format] being temporarily unavailable due to technical issues beyond our control.

BONUS

Guided Meditation Scripts for Mindful Eating: Nourishing Your Body and Soul.

Hello Mindful journeyer,

Welcome to a groundbreaking discussion — where the demonstration of eating rises above the everyday and turns into a sacrosanct custom. In the quick moving cadence of our lives, we frequently disregard the significant association between the food we eat and the sustenance it offers not exclusively to our bodies yet in addition to our spirits. You are invited to embark on a journey of self-discovery with this bonus content, "Guided Meditation Scripts for Mindful Eating," in which each bite becomes a mindful, intentional act of nourishing your body and soul.

Understanding Mindful Eating:

Before we dig into the directed reflection scripts, we should stop briefly to grasp the quintessence of careful eating. Mindful eating is certainly not a bunch of unbending principles or dietary limitations. All things considered, a workmanship — a training welcomes you to be completely present at the time, to enjoy the flavors, surfaces, and fragrances of your food, and to go with cognizant decisions about what and the amount you eat. It's tied in with developing a profound appreciation for the demonstration of eating and cultivating an agreeable relationship with the sustenance that supports you.

• The Benefits of Mindful Eating:

The advantages are complex. By embracing careful eating, you make the way for further developed processing, uplifted pleasure in food, better weight the executives, and expanded attention to your body's craving and completion prompts. A comprehensive methodology stretches out past actual sustenance, including mental and profound prosperity.

Let's take a look at the scripts for guided meditations that are meant to help you become more mindful while you eat.

Script 1: Preparation Meditation

Start by finding a tranquil space where you can sit easily. Shut your eyes and take a couple of full breaths. Look at the food in front of you as soon as you open your eyes. Permit your faculties to stir. Notice the varieties, surfaces, and smells. Offer thanks for the sustenance going to be gotten. Let this snapshot of readiness be a custom — an affirmation of the gift that supports you.

Script 2: Eating Awareness Meditation.

Change your focus to the act of eating. Take a nibble gradually and purposely. Shut your eyes as you relish the flavors moving on your sense of taste. Notice the temperature and surface of the food. Bite intentionally, permitting each chomp to unfurl its story. In the stops between nibbles, consider the tangible experience. Eating turns into an ensemble — a song of vibes that you are completely present to appreciate.

Script 3: Fullness and Satisfaction Reflection.

Halfway through your dinner, stop briefly for reflection. Check in with your body. How can it feel? Could it be said that you are fulfilled? Notice any signals of totality or satisfaction. This content aides you to come to careful conclusions about whether to keep eating or to respect your body's signs. It's a training in self-tuning in — an urgent part of careful eating.

Incorporating Mindful Eating into Daily Life:

As you explore these contents, consider how you can consistently incorporate careful eating into your day to day existence. Begin with one feast a day, steadily growing the training. Make a devoted eating space, liberated from interruptions, where every dinner turns into a sacrosanct snapshot of association. Create rituals that elevate the ordinary to the extraordinary.

Encouragement and Reflection:

Presently, we should finish up with a couple of inspirational statements. Embrace careful eating as an excursion — a continuous practice as opposed to an objective. Consider the potential benefits of this strategy for your relationship with food, overall health, and well-being. Keep in mind, each little, careful step you take adds to enduring change.

Your call to action:

Here is your source of inspiration: Coordinate these directed reflection scripts into your daily schedule. You'll find a connection to downloadable sound documents or a QR code for simple access. Take advantage of the practice and don't be afraid to talk about your challenges, insights, and experiences. Your excursion toward a more careful and deliberate way to deal with feasting begins now.

May your journey toward nourishing your body and soul be filled with mindfulness and joy, and may each bite be a celebration.

TABLE OF CONTENTS.

Introduction..**16**

Chapter 1..**20**

Understanding the Fundamentals.........................20

   • The Science of Metabolism........................... 20

   • How Your Burns Fat....................................22

   •The Role of Nutrition in Weight Management..24

Chapter 2..**29**

Unveiling the Dine Smart Principles...................... 29

   •Mindful Eating techniques.............................. 30

   •Balancing Macronutrients on Your Plate.........33

   •Portion Control Strategies............................. 35

Chapter 3..**39**

Superfoods for super results............................39

   •Exploring Nutrients-Rich Superfoods.............. 39

   • Recipes and Meal deals Featuring Superfoods.. 41

   •Incorporating Superfoods into Everyday Eating.. 42

Chapter 4..**46**

Smart strategies for sustainable weight loss.......... 46

   •Creating a personalized Meal Plan.................46

   • Tips for Healthy Snacking.............................48

   •Dining out without Derailing your Progress..... 50

Chapter 5..**54**

Exercise and Beyond...54

   • The role of physical activities in Weight Management.......................................54

• Building an Enjoyable Exercise Routine.........57

•Lifestyle Changes for Long term Success.......59

Chapter 6...**63**

Metabolism Boosters and Busters......................... 63

•Understanding Metabolism-boosting Habits....63

•Identifying and Overcoming Metabolism Blockers.. 66

•Practical Tips for Enhancing your Metabolism.68

Chapter 7...**71**

Aging Gracefully with Smart Nutrition.................... 71

•Nutritional Strategies For Longevity................ 71

•Foods that supports Healthy Aging................. 73

1. Vivid Berries:..73

• Anti-inflammatory Eating for joint Health........ 75

Chapter 8...**79**

Celebrating Your Wins... 79

•Tracking Progress and Celebrating Milestones... 79

•Maintaining Motivation For Continued Success.. 81

• Embracing a Life time of Smart Dining........... 83

Conclusion...**87**

• Reflecting on Your Journey................................87

•Empowered Eating for a Healthier, Happier You. 89

Introduction

Welcome To "Dine Smart, Win Big".

Permit me to tell you about a personal story that led to the creation of this guide. It was a journey that was filled with self-discovery, revelations about my health, and ultimately a commitment to change my life through mindful eating.

Quite a long while back, my relationship with food was wild, best case scenario. I swayed between snapshots of extravagance, appreciating the kinds of life, and times of culpability loaded endeavors at prohibitive weight control plans.

This cycle left me feeling genuinely depleted, actually exhausted, and frequently crushed by my own desires.

•The Connection Between Nutrition and Overall Health

My perspective dramatically changed during a seemingly ordinary day's routine checkup. A progression of blood tests and a sincere discussion with my PCP uncovered the irrefutable connection between my dietary propensities and the condition of my wellbeing. My body, when a latent member in my culinary experiences, arose as a perplexing framework that blossomed with sustenance as opposed to simple utilization.

The disclosure was both alarming and engaging. I started to perceive that each piece I ingested conveyed outcomes a long way past the quick joy it gave. Sustenance wasn't just about calories; It had an impact on energy levels, mental clarity, and resistance to illness, making it the foundation of overall well-being.

•Setting the stage for a successful Journey.

Persuaded by newly discovered mindfulness, I set out on an excursion to "Feast Shrewd, Win Large." This guide is definitely not a simple gathering of dietary realities; it's a demonstration of the examples I gathered through experimentation. It's tied in with making way for a fruitful and practical excursion towards wellbeing and satisfaction.

"Eat Shrewd, Win Large" is established in the conviction that genuine change isn't found in drastic actions however in the careful, ordinary decisions we make. Through sharing my own story, I expect to associate with you on a more profound level, offering a brief look into the difficulties, wins, and examples that prepared me for a more adjusted and satisfying life.

Thus, as we leave on this excursion together, how about we turn each page with the comprehension that each feast is a chance for positive change. This book isn't simply counsel; it's a friend in your quest for a day to day existence where eating savvy implies winning huge. Here's to the pages ahead — may they be as extraordinary for you as they have been for me.

Chapter 1.

Understanding the Fundamentals.

Welcome to Section 1 of our excursion together: Today, we're going to look at the intricate world of metabolism, how your body burns fat, and the crucial role nutrition plays in weight management. Thus, get some tea or espresso, track down a comfortable spot, and we should leave on this edifying discussion.

• The Science of Metabolism

To understand digestion, we should envision your body as a clamoring city. The occupants of this city are cells, and the energy they expect to work is produced by metabolic cycles. Digestion includes a progression of substance responses inside these cells that convert the food you eat into the energy expected to support life.

1. **Anabolic and catabolic metabolism:**

At its center, digestion comprises two key cycles — anabolism and catabolism. The use of energy in anabolism is required for the creation of complex molecules from simpler ones. Catabolism, then again, is the breakdown of perplexing particles into less difficult ones, delivering energy.

2. **Energy Money - ATP:**

Adenosine Triphosphate (ATP) is the energy cash of the cell. Consider ATP to be the coins that power our city's various functions. Through cell breath, our cells remove energy from supplements, basically glucose, and convert it into ATP.

3. **Factors Impacting Metabolism:**

While hereditary qualities assume a part in deciding your gauge digestion, way of life factors like eating routine, active work, and try and rest can fundamentally influence it. Standard activity, for example, consumes calories during the action as well as raises your resting metabolic rate, permitting you to consume more calories even very still.

It is not enough to simply classify metabolism as "fast" or "slow." It's a dynamic, versatile framework, similar to the city changing its speed in view of the requests of its occupants.

• How Your Burns Fat

Presently, how about we adventure into the entrancing universe of fat digestion — the ballistic course of putting away and using fat for energy.

1. The Fat Stockpiling Myth:
In opposition to mainstream thinking, fat isn't the enemy; it's an indispensable energy hold. At the point when you consume a bigger number of calories than your body requires, the

overabundance is put away as fat. This capacity is an endurance system, giving a wellspring of energy during times of shortage.

2. Getting Lipolysis Started:

Lipolysis starts when your body needs more energy than it has from the food you've eaten. This interaction includes separating put away fat into unsaturated fats and glycerol. These parts are then shipped through the circulation system, where they can be used for energy through an interaction called beta-oxidation.

3. Act of balancing:

Powerful weight the board isn't tied in with taking out fat yet rather finding some kind of harmony. Accomplishing a feasible and sound weight includes coordinating this dance between fat capacity and use. It's tied in with establishing a climate wherein your body effectively takes advantage of its fat stores when required.

•The Role of Nutrition in Weight Management

Now that we have a solid understanding of the fundamentals of metabolism and fat burning, let's turn our attention to the significant influence that nutrition has on weight management.

1. Past Calorie Counting:

While the principle of calories in versus calories out is fundamental to weight management, it is essential to go beyond counting calories. The nature of those calories matters monstrously. Envision your body as a finely tuned machine — furnishing it with the right blend of macronutrients (starches, proteins, and fats) and micronutrients (nutrients and minerals) guarantees ideal working.

2. Carbohydrates:

Carbs, frequently misjudged, are your body's favored wellspring of energy. The key is to choose complex carbohydrates over refined sugars, which are found in whole grains, fruits, and vegetables. The previous gives a supported arrival of energy, forestalling insulin spikes that can prompt fat stockpiling.

3. Proteins:

Proteins are the structure blocks of tissues and assume a critical part in the weight the board. Remembering satisfactory protein for your eating regimen not just guides in satiety, diminishing the probability of gorging, yet additionally upholds muscle safeguarding during weight reduction.

4. Fats:

Fats, frequently attacked, are fundamental for different physical processes. Select sound fats tracked down in avocados, nuts, and olive oil, as they add to chemical creation, supplement retention, and mind capability.

5. Micronutrients:

In weight management, micronutrients like vitamins and minerals are the unsung heroes. Inadequacies can disturb metabolic cycles, underscoring the significance of a balanced eating routine that incorporates various supplement thick food varieties.

6. Individual Variability:

It's vital to recognize that there's nobody size-fits-all way to deal with nourishment. Each body is one of a kind, answering diversely to different dietary examples. The excursion includes self-disclosure — tuning into your body's signs, trying different things with various wholesome systems, and finding what lines up with your singular requirements and objectives.

As we finish up this discussion of chapter 1, think about the interconnectedness of these essential ideas. Your body is a dynamic, versatile framework, and the decisions with respect to food and way of life are the strings that weave the complicated embroidery of your wellbeing.

Thus, dear companion, outfitted with a more profound comprehension of digestion, fat consuming, and the job of sustenance in weight the executives, you have the information to settle on informed decisions. This journey is a partnership in which you and your body cooperate to communicate, adjust, and thrive.

Chapter 2

Unveiling the Dine Smart Principles.

Today, we leave on an excursion to change the manner in which you approach dinners. We'll investigate careful eating methods, talk about the craft of adjusting macronutrients on your plate, and dive into powerful part control procedures. Thus, how about we step into this domain of cognizant feasting and disentangle the rules that can reclassify your relationship with food.

•Mindful Eating techniques.

Envision a feast as in excess of a simple assortment of supplements — it's an encounter, a second to relish, appreciate, and sustain your body as well as your spirit. This is what mindful eating is all about.

1. Drawing in the Senses:

Engaging your senses is the first step in eating mindfully. Prior to taking that first nibble, pause for a minute to notice the varieties, surfaces, and smells of your food. Permit your faculties to drench themselves in the culinary experience completely.

2. Relishing Each Bite:

In our quick moving world, it's not difficult to race through dinners without really tasting them. Careful eating urges you to enjoy each nibble, appreciating the flavors and surfaces. Allow yourself to fully experience eating by putting your utensils down between bites.

3. Paying attention to Your Body:

Your body imparts its necessities, yet the racket of current life frequently muffles these signs. Careful eating includes checking out your body's yearning and completion signals. Eat when you're eager, stop when you're fulfilled, and perceive the inconspicuous signs that demonstrate your body's prerequisites.

4. Disposing of Distractions:

Picture a quiet eating experience — no TV, no cell phone, just you and your feast. Limiting interruptions during dinners permits you to be available, encouraging a more profound association with your food and advancing careful utilization.

5. Appreciation and Awareness:

Gratitude for the food you eat should be expressed. Know about the work that went into delivering your food, from ranch to table. The act of eating becomes a mindful ritual as a result of this shift in perspective.

Mindful eating is a training, an excursion of developing mindfulness and cultivating an agreeable relationship with the food you eat. It transforms each meal into a celebration of joy and sustenance and is an invitation to be completely present in the moment.

•Balancing Macronutrients on Your Plate.

The thought of a decent feast reaches out past assortment; it includes understanding and integrating the fundamental macronutrients — carbs, proteins, and fats — into your day to day diet.

1. Carbohydrates:

Frequently depicted as the lowlife in some eating routine stories, sugars are your body's essential wellspring of energy. For sustained energy release, choose complex carbohydrates found in whole grains, fruits, and vegetables. Consider them the underpinning of your dinner.

2. Proteins:

Proteins are the structure blocks of life, adding to the design and capability of tissues. Remembering satisfactory protein for your eating routine advances satiety, helps with muscle fix, and supports different physiological capabilities. Settle on lean sources like poultry, fish, vegetables, and tofu.

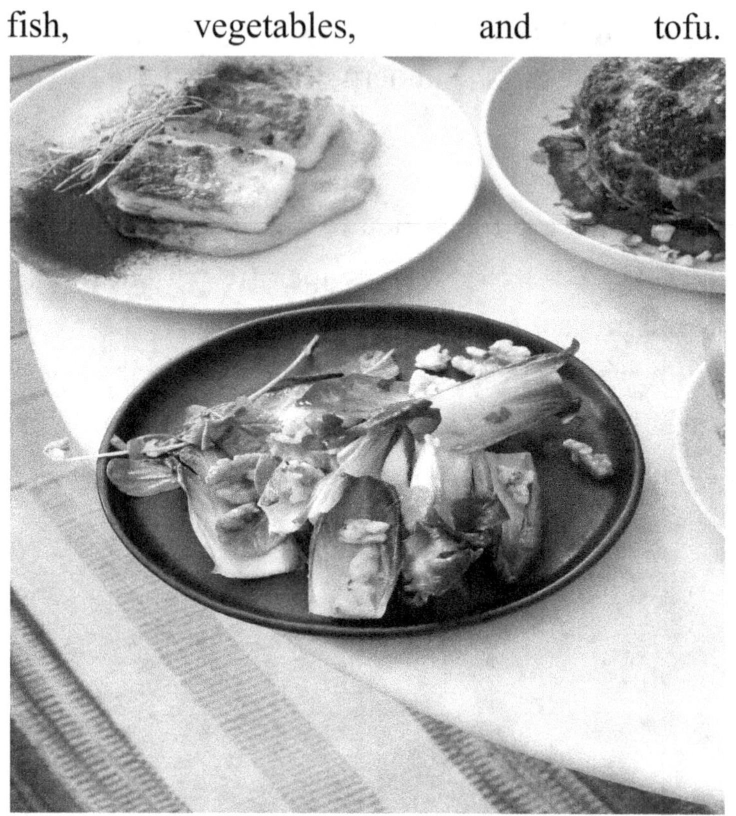

3. Fats:

Solid fats are fundamental for generally speaking prosperity. They assume a part in chemical creation, supplement retention, and even mind wellbeing. Consolidate wellsprings of solid fats, similar to avocados, nuts, seeds, and olive oil, into your feasts. Balance is critical — appreciate them with some restraint.

4. The Concordance of Colors:

Picture your plate as a material, and the shades of your food as the range. Hold back nothing scope of varieties, as various tints frequently mean unmistakable wholesome profiles. This not just improves the visual allure of your dinner yet additionally guarantees a wide range of supplements.

•Portion Control Strategies.

In this present reality where "supersize" segments have turned into the standard, excelling at segment control is an expertise that can significantly influence your wellbeing.

1. Careful Serving Sizes:

Start by rethinking your view of serving sizes. It's not difficult to misjudge the sum we eat, particularly when confronted with liberal bits. Utilize viewable signs, for example, contrasting your protein segment with the size of your palm, to direct your serving sizes.

2. More modest Plates and Bowls:

Your perception of portion sizes may be influenced by the size of your dishware. Settle on more modest plates and bowls, making a deception of overflow with more modest measures of food. This straightforward stunt can assist with managing your bits without leaving you feeling denied.

3. Pay attention to Yearning Cues:

Check out your body's signs. Inquire as to whether you're genuinely eager or on the other hand on the off chance that you're eating without much forethought, weariness, or stress. Answering certifiable craving signs permits you to adjust your eating designs with your body's requirements.

4. Pre-Dividing and Feast Planning:

Assume command over your parts by pre-parceling dinners and bites. This can be especially useful with food sources that are not difficult to gorge. Having a meal plan also gives you structure and makes it easier to choose what to eat and how much to eat.

5. Hydration:

Now and again, what we see as yearning is really thirst. Remain hydrated over the course of the day, and prior to going after a tidbit, stop and look at whether a glass of water would fulfill your body's necessities.

Segment control isn't about hardship however about finding the offset that lines up with your body's necessities. It's a way of life that lets you savor the pleasures of eating while honoring your body's signals of fullness.

As we close this discussion of chapter 2, consider the extraordinary power these standards hold. Balanced macronutrients, mindful eating, and effective portion control aren't rules; rather, they are tools that empower you to have a healthier, more conscious relationship with food.

May your excursion through these standards be loaded up with self-disclosure, sustenance, and a recently discovered appreciation for the craft of feasting shrewd.

Chapter 3.

Superfoods for super results.

Hi Inquisitive Personalities,Welcome to Section 3.

Here, we're wandering into the domain of supplement stuffed superfoods, investigating how they can lift your nourishment, offering food as well as a heap of medical advantages. Thus, lock in for an excursion into the universe of lively varieties, novel flavors, and super outcomes.

•Exploring Nutrients-Rich Superfoods

1. Grasping Superfoods:

Superfoods are nourishing forces to be reckoned with, thickly loaded with nutrients, minerals, cancer prevention agents, and other fundamental supplements. These foods have numerous health-enhancing properties that go beyond basic nutrition.

2. Various Superfood Options:

The universe of superfoods is brilliantly assorted. From the natural, like berries and mixed greens, to the intriguing, such as acai berries and spirulina, there's a superfood to suit each sense of taste. Each offers a one of a kind supplement profile that might be of some value, adding to by and large prosperity.

3. Cancer prevention agent Richness:

The high antioxidant content of many superfoods has made them famous. Cancer prevention agents battle oxidative pressure in the body, safeguarding cells from harm. Berries, dull mixed greens, and nuts are amazing models, exhibiting the lively varieties that frequently signal cancer prevention agent intensity.

• Recipes and Meal deals Featuring Superfoods.

1. Superfood Smoothie Bowl:

A smoothie bowl filled with superfoods is a great way to start the day. Blend chia seeds, spinach, frozen berries, and a little almond milk together. Top it with cut kiwi, granola, and a sprinkle of cell reinforcement rich goji berries.

2. Quinoa and Kale Salad:

Hoist your lunch with a quinoa and kale salad. Throw cooked quinoa with hacked kale, cherry tomatoes, avocado, and a shower of olive oil. This thick plate of mixed greens is an ideal equilibrium of protein, sound fats, and nutrients.

3. Salmon with Turmeric and Ginger:

Consolidate superfoods into your supper by getting ready salmon prepared with turmeric and ginger. These flavors, celebrated for their calming properties, add flavor as well as add to the dish's superfood status.

•Incorporating Superfoods into Everyday Eating.

1.Begin Small:

If the universe of superfoods feels overpowering, begin little. Present each new superfood in turn, permitting your taste buds and body to change. The gradual introduction of superfoods into your diet makes them easier to maintain over time.

2. Blend and Match:

Embrace the excellence of assortment. Blend and match different superfoods to make a vivid and supplement rich plate. The more assorted your superfood admission, the more extensive the range of supplements you give your body.

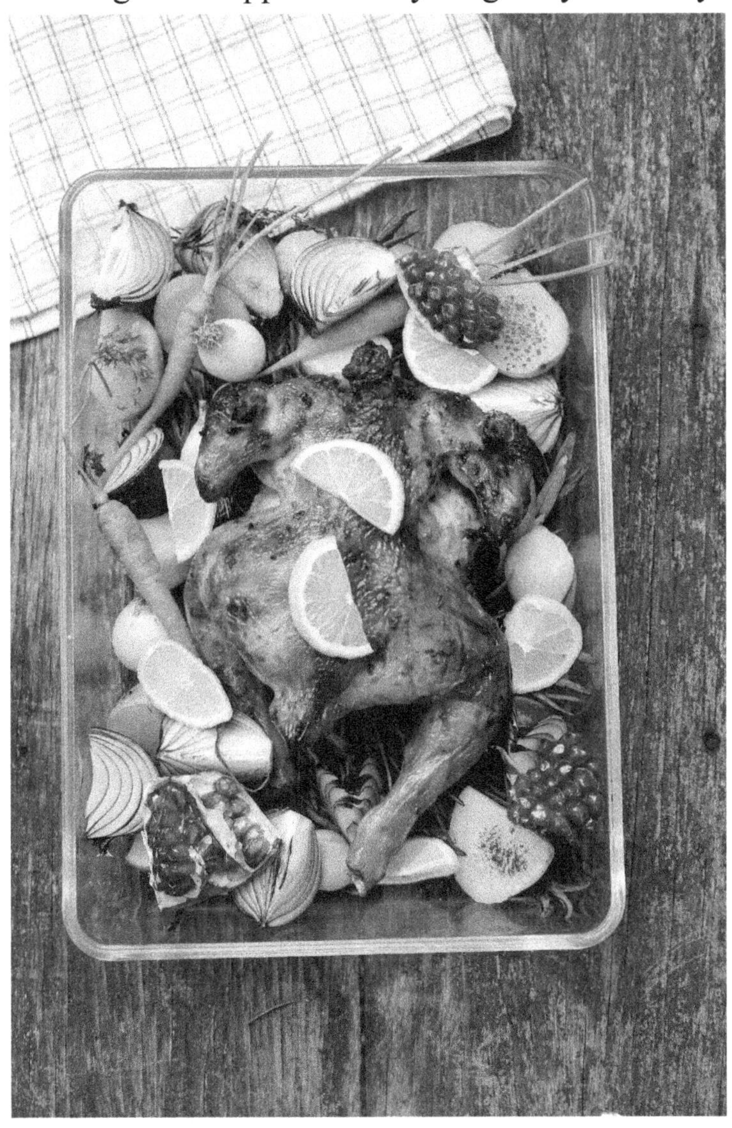

3. Superfood Snacking:

Change your snacks into nourishing forces to be reckoned with. Snatch a modest bunch of blended nuts, a serving of Greek yogurt with berries, or crunchy kale chips for a superfood-imbued jolt of energy.

In the woven artwork of your everyday dinners, superfoods add lively shades and multifaceted examples. They are not merely components; they're the structure blocks of a better, more sustained you.

As we wrap up this discussion of Section 3, consider the little, deliberate advances you can take to imbue your dinners with superfood goodness. There's no need to focus on sensational changes yet about embracing the capability of these supplement rich marvels to upgrade your general prosperity.

May your culinary experiences with superfoods be both delightful and groundbreaking.

Chapter 4

Smart strategies for sustainable weight loss.

Welcome to Chapter 4, fellow wellness enthusiasts.

In this part, we'll explore the territory of customized feast arranging, find the craft of solid eating, and unwind the mysteries of feasting out without undermining your advancement. Thus, we should set out on this excursion toward supportable weight reduction, where each decision is a stage toward a better, more joyful you.

•Creating a personalized Meal Plan

1. Recognizing Your Needs.

The groundwork of a customized dinner plan lies in figuring out your remarkable dietary necessities. Factors, for example, age, movement level, digestion, and wellbeing objectives assume a significant part. Talking with a sustenance expert can give significant bits of knowledge, yet natural mindfulness is similarly urgent.

2. Adjusting Macronutrients:

A balanced dinner plan includes an equilibrium of macronutrients — carbs, proteins, and fats. Tailor these extents in view of your singular necessities. For example, assuming that you take part in normal actual work, changing your protein admission to help muscle recuperation might be valuable.

3. Entire Food varieties Emphasis:

Focus on supplementing thick food sources in your dinner plan. These incorporate natural products, vegetables, lean proteins, entire grains, and sound fats. Entire food sources give fundamental supplements as well as add to a feeling of completion and fulfillment.

4. Feast Timing and Frequency:

Think about the timing and recurrence of your dinners. While some individuals benefit from smaller, more frequent meals, others thrive on three large meals per day. Pay attention to your body's appetite and satiety signs to figure out what dinner timing suits you best.

• Tips for Healthy Snacking.

1. Careful Snacking:

The enemy is not snacking; it's an amazing chance to support your body between dinners. Embrace careful nibbling by picking supplement rich choices. New natural product, Greek yogurt, a small bunch of nuts, or vegetable sticks with hummus are fulfilling and healthy decisions.

2. The key is preparation:

To avoid reaching for less nutritious options when hunger strikes, plan your snacks in advance. Having pre-cut veggies, parceled nuts, or a piece of natural product promptly accessible makes sound eating more helpful.

3. Hydration:

Sometimes, what appears to be thirst is actually hunger. Remain hydrated over the course of the day, and when a tidbit hankering hits, think about going after a glass of water first. It very well may be exactly what your body needs.

4. Protein-Stuffed Options:

Snacking on protein can help you feel fuller longer and help keep your muscles healthy. Protein-rich options include a few edamame, a small serving of cottage cheese, or hard-boiled eggs.

•Dining out without Derailing your Progress.

1. Careful Menu Exploration:

While eating out, move toward the menu as an open door instead of a test. Search for dishes that integrate lean proteins, different vegetables, and entire grains. Numerous cafés now highlight better choices, frequently indicated on the menu.

2. Awareness of portions:

Café segments are frequently bigger than whatever you could serve at home. Be aware of piece estimates, and consider imparting dishes to feasting partners or pressing portion of your dinner to-go before you even beginning eating.

3. Smarter Alternatives:

Don't hesitate for even a moment to modify your request. Request dressings or sauces on the side, choose grilled rather than fried, and substitute fries for a side salad. These little replacements can fundamentally influence the generally wholesome substance of your feast.

4. Pay attention to your body:

Focus on your body's signals while eating out. Eat gradually, appreciate each chomp, and stop when you feel fulfilled. Keep in mind, it's entirely satisfactory to bring extras back home — view it as a little something extra dinner for the following day.

• **Embracing Manageability in Your Weight reduction Excursion**.

1. Consistency Over Perfection:

Maintainable weight reduction isn't about flawlessness yet about consistency. Go for the gold, flawlessness. Little, slow changes are bound to become enduring propensities than exceptional, momentary measures.

2. Building a healthy connection to food:

Shift your point of view toward food as sustenance instead of a wellspring of responsibility or limitation. A positive relationship with food includes getting a charge out of dinners, embracing various flavors, and commending the sustenance your decisions give.

3. Regular sports participation:

Supplement your dietary endeavors with normal actual work. Find types of activity you appreciate, whether it's strolling, moving, or weightlifting. Physical activity not only helps people lose weight, but it also improves their overall health.

4. Adjusting to Changing Needs:

Your body's necessities advance over the long haul. Be available to changing your feast plan and way of life to oblige these changes. What worked for you in one period of your process might require change as you progress.

As we come to the end of this study of Chapter 4, keep in mind that long-term weight loss requires a holistic approach. It involves more than just what you eat; it also involves how you prepare meals, snacks, and outings. About making a way of life upholds your wellbeing and prosperity, each careful decision in turn.

Welcome to the journey toward long-term weight loss, a journey in which every step forward should be celebrated.

Chapter 5.

Exercise and Beyond.

Dear Wellness Lovers, Welcome to chapter 5.
This portion of our process dives into the necessary job of actual work in weight, the executives, guides you in building an agreeable work-out daily practice, and investigates way of life changes urgent for long haul achievement. In this way, we should bind up those shoes and embrace the all encompassing way to deal with wellbeing and prosperity.

• The role of physical activities in Weight Management.

1. Past Caloric Burn:

While the caloric consumption of activity is evidently a calculated weight of the board, its effect goes past simple numbers. Ordinary actual work impacts digestion, further develops insulin awareness, and supports the protection of slender bulk. Because of its multiple functions, exercise is an essential component of long-term weight management.

2. Boost in metabolism:

Your metabolic rate can be increased by participating in both aerobic and resistance training. Cardiovascular activities like running, swimming, or cycling raise your pulse, expanding calorie consumption during the movement and possibly prompting an "afterburn" impact, where the body keeps on consuming calories post-work out. Opposition preparing, then again, assembles muscle, which is metabolically dynamic and adds to long haul metabolic wellbeing.

3. Hormonal Balance:

Physical activity is important for weight management because it affects hormonal balance. Exercise can upgrade the arrival of endorphins, diminishing pressure and profound eating. It also regulates hormones like insulin and cortisol, which helps to improve fat metabolism and improve energy balance.

4. Craving Regulation:

Customary active work has been displayed to assist with directing craving. It can impact chemicals like ghrelin and leptin, which assume key parts in yearning and satiety. A very much planned work-out routine can make a positive input circle, where active work upholds hunger control, making it more straightforward to stick to a reasonable eating regimen.

• Building an Enjoyable Exercise Routine.

1. Finding Your Preferences:

Practice shouldn't feel like a task; it ought to be a pleasant piece of your daily practice. Investigate various sorts of active work to find what impacts you. Whether it's moving, climbing, weightlifting, or yoga, finding exercises you really appreciate improves the probability of consistency.

2. Realistic Objectives:

Lay out reasonable and reachable wellness objectives. Whether it's finishing a 5K, dominating another yoga present, or expanding your weightlifting limit, setting achievements provides your work-out routine motivation and inspiration. Commend these accomplishments, regardless of how little — they are venturing stones toward long haul achievement.

3. Assortment and Adaptability:

By including a variety of exercises, you can keep your routine fresh. This ensures a comprehensive fitness strategy in addition to avoiding monotony. Include activities that improve balance and coordination as well as cardiovascular workouts, strength training, and flexibility exercises.

4. Social Engagement:

Think about making exercise a party. Whether it's joining a gathering wellness class, tracking down an exercise pal, or partaking in group activities, the social viewpoint can change practice into a tomfoolery and local area driven insight. The brotherhood and backing can make the excursion more agreeable and manageable.

5. Connection between the Mind and the Body:

Develop a mindful exercise routine. Focus on how your body feels during and after active work. This mindfulness can assist you with fitting your daily practice to line up with your body's requirements, cultivating a positive relationship with work.

•Lifestyle Changes for Long term Success

1. Consistency Over Intensity:

Long haul progress in weight the executives is based on consistency as opposed to outrageous power. Feasible way of life changes include pursuing decisions that you can keep up with after some time. This could mean selecting a moderate work-out schedule that you truly appreciate and tracking down a reasonable way to deal with sustenance.

2. Sleep and Managing Stress:

Recognize the effect of rest and weight on weight the executives. Quality rest is fundamental for hormonal guideline and generally prosperity. Carry out pressure the executives procedures like care, contemplation, or side interests to establish a strong climate for your wellbeing objectives.

3. Fuel from Food:

View nourishment as fuel for your body instead of a prohibitive arrangement of rules. Embrace a reasonable and differed diet that upholds your energy needs. Center around entire, supplement thick food sources, and be aware of piece sizes. Take a stab at a practical methodology that permits adaptability and happiness in your dietary patterns.

4. Careful Eating Practices:

Integrate careful eating rehearses into your way of life. Focus on appetite and completion signs, enjoy the kinds of your feasts, and limit interruptions during eating. Careful eating not just adds to a better relationship with food yet additionally upholds weight the board by advancing cognizant utilization.

5. Adjusting to Life Changes:

Life is dynamic, thus ought to be your way to deal with wellbeing. Be able to change with life, whether it's your career, family, or personal milestones. Your work-out everyday practice and nourishment plan ought to advance with you, guaranteeing they stay sensible and economical in various periods of life.

Fundamentally, "Exercise and Beyond" implies a comprehensive point of view on wellbeing. It's not just about consuming calories; about developing a way of life supports your body, brain, and soul.

Chapter 6

Metabolism Boosters and Busters.

Welcome to Chapter 6, Health Enthusiasts.

In this section, we'll unwind the secrets of digestion, investigating propensities that give it a lift, distinguishing possible blockers, and offering functional tips to improve this crucial cycle. Therefore, let's discuss the intricate world of metabolism and equip ourselves with information that will shape our health journey.

•Understanding Metabolism-boosting Habits.

1. The Establishment: Healthy Eating:

At the center of a digestion supporting way of life lies adjusted nourishment. Giving your body the right blend of macronutrients — carbs, proteins, and fats — guarantees ideal energy creation. Entire, supplement thick food sources contribute not exclusively to satiety yet additionally to the proficiency of metabolic cycles.

2. Regular sports participation:

Practice is a strong digestion promoter. Both cardiovascular exercises, like running or cycling, and obstruction preparing, such as weightlifting, add to expanded calorie consumption. The beneficial outcomes reach out past the exercise, as normal active work can hoist your resting metabolic rate.

3. Hydration for Ideal Function:

Remaining enough hydrated is a basic yet frequently disregarded digestion supporter. Water is engaged with various metabolic cycles, and lack of hydration can prevent the proficiency of these capabilities. Practice it all the time to taste water over the course of the day to help your body's metabolic apparatus.

4. Training in Intervals for Afterburn:

Intense cardio exercise (HIIT) is prestigious for its capacity to help digestion. The short eruptions of extreme movement followed by brief reprieve periods consume calories during the exercise as well as actuate an afterburn impact, where the body keeps on consuming calories post-work out.

5. Satisfactory Rest for Hormonal Harmony:

Quality rest is a digestion partner. Absence of rest disturbs hormonal equilibrium, influencing hunger controlling chemicals like ghrelin and leptin. Hold back nothing long stretches of value rest each night to help your body's metabolic amicability.

•Identifying and Overcoming Metabolism Blockers.

1. Inactive Lifestyle:

Delayed times of idleness can dial back digestion. Whether it's because of a work area work or an absence of active work, battle an inactive way of life by integrating development into your day. Stand up routinely, go for short strolls, or think about a standing work area to keep your body moving.

2.   Crash Diets and Outrageous Caloric Restriction:

Crash diets and outrageous caloric limitation can blow up on digestion. In order to conserve energy, the body goes into a state of conservation when it perceives a severe lack of food. Select a decent, economical way to deal with nourishment that upholds your energy needs.

3. Absence of Protein in Diet:

Protein assumes an essential part in keeping up with bulk, and muscle is metabolically dynamic tissue. Your body's capacity to maintain a healthy metabolic rate may be compromised if you consume insufficient protein in your diet. Incorporate lean protein sources like poultry, fish, tofu, and vegetables in your feasts.

4. Stress and Cortisol Impact:

Constant pressure can raise cortisol levels, which might add to metabolic brokenness.

Consolidate pressure the executives practices like contemplation, profound breathing, or yoga into your daily schedule. Focus on taking care of oneself to establish a fair and strong climate for your digestion.

5. Lacking Hydration:

Drying out dials back metabolic cycles as well as influences your body's capacity to productively use energy. Make sure you drink enough water every day and think about including foods that hydrate you, like fruits and vegetables, in your diet.

•Practical Tips for Enhancing your Metabolism.

1. Eat a variety of meals throughout the day:

Rather than a couple of huge dinners, think about spreading your feasts over the course of the day. This methodology, known as touching or eating more modest, more incessant dinners, can assist with keeping a consistent progression of energy and backing metabolic capability.

2. Consolidate Flavors and Green Tea:

Certain flavors, for example, cayenne pepper, and drinks like green tea, have been related with an impermanent expansion in metabolic rate. While the impact might be unassuming, integrating these into your eating regimen can add a delightful lift to your digestion.

3. Creating and Keeping Muscle Mass:

Muscle is metabolically dynamic tissue, meaning it consumes a bigger number of calories very still than fat. Take part in opposition preparing to assemble and keep up with bulk. This supports a solid digestion as well as adds to generally speaking strength and prosperity.

4. Get Your Omega-3s:

Omega-3 unsaturated fats, tracked down in greasy fish, flaxseeds, and pecans, have been connected to worked on metabolic wellbeing. Remembering wellsprings of omega-3s for your eating regimen upholds cell capability and can decidedly impact metabolic cycles.

5. Careful Eating Practices:

Develop careful dietary patterns. Focus on craving and totality signals, enjoy the kinds of your feasts, and limit interruptions during eating. Mindful eating encourages conscious consumption, which helps maintain a healthy metabolism and prevents overeating.

Wishing you a digestion loaded up with energy and dynamic quality.

Chapter 7

Aging Gracefully with Smart Nutrition.

Hi Wise Spirits,Welcome to Chapter 7.In this part, we'll explore nourishment methodologies for life span, uncover food varieties that help solid maturing, and dive into the domain of mitigating eating for joint wellbeing. Maturing is a characteristic piece of life, and through savvy sustenance, we can embrace this excursion with beauty, imperativeness, and insight.

•Nutritional Strategies For Longevity

1. Plant-Based Embrace:

Embracing a plant-based diet is a foundation of nourishment for life span. Plant-based food sources, wealthy in cell reinforcements, fiber, and a variety of micronutrients, add to in general prosperity. Try to eat a wide range of colorful fruits, vegetables, whole grains, nuts, and legumes on your plate.

2. Calorie Mindful Intake:

As we age, our digestion might dial back, making it significant to be aware of caloric admission. Center around supplement thick food varieties that give fundamental nutrients and minerals without abundance calories. Focus on higher expectations without ever compromising to meet your body's evolving needs.

3. Protein for Muscle Maintenance:

Protein turns out to be progressively significant with age, supporting muscle upkeep and generally essentialness. Incorporate lean protein sources like fish, poultry, tofu, and vegetables in your dinners. Disseminate protein consumption over the course of the day to upgrade muscle combination.

4. Fundamental Greasy Acids:

Include sources of essential fatty acids in your diet, particularly omega-3s. These fats, tracked down in greasy fish, flaxseeds, and pecans, have calming properties and backing cerebrum wellbeing. Including them in your diet helps you live longer in a holistic way.

•Foods that supports Healthy Aging.

1. Vivid Berries:

Berries, like blueberries, strawberries, and raspberries, are wealthy in cell reinforcements that battle oxidative pressure — a vital consider maturing. These energetic natural products likewise give fiber, advancing stomach related wellbeing and adding to generally prosperity.

2. Verdant Greens:

Powerhouses of nutrients are dark leafy greens like Swiss chard, spinach, and kale. Loaded with nutrients, minerals, and cancer prevention agents, they support resistant capability, bone wellbeing, and may add to mental prosperity.

3. Nuts and Seeds:

Nuts and seeds are supplement thick bites that offer an abundance of medical advantages.

Almonds, pecans, chia seeds, and flaxseeds give omega-3 unsaturated fats, fiber, and different nutrients and minerals. They're advantageous increments to dinners or wonderful all alone.

4. Crunchy Fish:

Omega-3 fatty acids can be found in abundance in fatty fish like salmon, mackerel, and sardines. These fats have been related with a diminished gamble of persistent illnesses and may uphold heart and mind wellbeing as we age.

5. Entire Grains:

Entire grains like quinoa, earthy colored rice, and oats give fundamental supplements, including fiber and complex carbs. These grains help maintain energy levels and support digestive health, both of which contribute to longevity.

• Anti-inflammatory Eating for joint Health.

1.Turmeric and Curcumin:

Turmeric, a flavor frequently found in curry dishes, contains curcumin, known for its mitigating properties. Integrate turmeric into your cooking or consider taking curcumin supplements, with direction from a medical services proficient, to help joint wellbeing.

2. Omega-3-Rich Foods:

Omega-3 fatty acids, which can be found in flaxseeds, chia seeds, and fatty fish, reduce inflammation. If you eat these foods, you might be able to lower inflammation, which will help your joints and overall health.

3. Brilliant Vegetables:

Vivid vegetables, especially those with a profound tint like peppers, tomatoes, and carrots, are wealthy in cell reinforcements. These cell reinforcements battle irritation and backing joint wellbeing. Hold back nothing exhibit of veggies to amplify their healthful advantages.

4. Ginger:

Ginger has for quite some time been adulated for its mitigating properties. Whether utilized in teas, added to dishes, or taken as an enhancement, ginger might add to decreasing irritation and easing joint uneasiness.

5. Green Tea:

Green tea is eminent for its high convergence of polyphenols, which have mitigating and cancer prevention agent impacts. Partake in some green tea as a component of your everyday daily schedule to advance joint wellbeing and by and large prosperity.

• Embracing Aging as an Excursion.

Improving with age isn't just about the years we aggregate however the personal satisfaction we keep up with. We can use smart nutrition as a compass to help us survive and thrive on this journey. As we investigate systems for life span, we should recollect that maturing is an honor denied to many, and every day presents a chance to put resources into our prosperity.

May your way be decorated with the shades of sustenance, insight, and the hug of each passing season.

Chapter 8.

Celebrating Your Wins.

Welcome to Part 8.In this section, we'll leave on an excursion of self-reflection and affirmation, investigating the significance of following advancement, commending achievements, keeping up with inspiration for proceeded with progress, and embracing a long period of savvy eating. Life is a progression of triumphs, and each step in the right direction should be perceived and celebrated.

•Tracking Progress and Celebrating Milestones.

1. Setting Clear Goals:

The groundwork of progress following lies in setting clear, feasible objectives. Whether your targets are connected with weight reduction, wellness, or by and large prosperity, characterizing explicit, quantifiable, and sensible objectives gives a guide to your excursion.

2. Using Technology:

Embrace the force of innovation to keep tabs on your development. You can evaluate your journey objectively by using fitness apps, nutrition trackers, and wearable devices that provide valuable insights into your daily routines. Consistently survey your information to recognize designs, praise accomplishments, and make informed changes.

3. Journaling Your Journey:

Past numbers, consider journaling your encounters. Record how you feel subsequent to accomplishing a wellness achievement, conquering a dietary test, or dominating another sound propensity. Your personal story adds depth to your journey and motivates you through both highs and lows.

4. Dreaming of Success:

Make a visual portrayal of your advancement. Whether it's a dream board, a chart following your weight reduction venture, or a photograph journal displaying your wellness accomplishments, obvious signals act as strong tokens of how far you've come.

•Maintaining Motivation For Continued Success.

1. Thinking about Your "Why":

Return to the purposes for your wellbeing and health venture. Think about the inherent inspirations — further developed energy, upgraded prosperity, or expanded self-assurance — that filled your underlying responsibility. Interfacing with your "why" revives the enthusiasm pushing you forward.

2. Changing Objectives as Needed:

Be willing to adjust your objectives as your journey progresses. Life is dynamic, and your yearnings might advance. Whether you're arriving at an objective sooner than anticipated or recalibrating in light of evolving conditions, adaptable objective setting guarantees proceeded with inspiration.

3. Developing a Help System:

Begin your journey with a community that will support you. Whether it's companions, family, or individual health fans, a steady organization gives consolation during difficulties and offers in the delight of your victories. Celebrate achievements together and draw strength from aggregate inspiration.

4. Compensating Yourself Thoughtfully:

Consider executing smart awards for arriving at achievements. Food-based rewards are not required; they could be encounters, taking care of oneself ceremonies, or things that line up with your prosperity. Smart prizes support positive way of behaving and add to supported inspiration.

5. Investigating New Challenges:

Battle lack of concern by presenting new difficulties. Whether it's difficult an alternate exercise, trying different things with new solid recipes, or investigating a wellness class, oddity flashes fervor and forestalls repetitiveness. Embracing difficulties encourages a mentality of nonstop development.

• Embracing a Life time of Smart Dining

1. Making Maintainable Habits:

Brilliant eating isn't about prohibitive weight control plans however about making supportable propensities. Embrace a reasonable way to deal with nourishment that considers happiness while focusing on wellbeing. Manageability guarantees that your eating decisions add to a long period of prosperity.

2. Eating intuitively:

Develop instinctive dietary patterns. Pay attention to your body's yearning and completion signals, and focus on how various food sources cause you to feel. Regarding your body's signs encourages a careful and positive relationship with food.

3. Adjusting Indulgences:

Shrewd eating doesn't mean total evasion of extravagances. Balance is critical. Partake in your #1 treats with some restraint, enjoying the experience without responsibility. This fair methodology makes your health process feasible and pleasant.

4. Feast Anticipating Success:

Include meal preparation into your daily routine. Arranging feasts ahead of time permits you to make purposeful, nutritious decisions. It likewise assists you with opposing the enticement of unfortunate choices when confronted with unconstrained feasting choices.

• The Specialty of celebration

Commending your successes is a craftsmanship — an orchestra of self-acknowledgment, appreciation, and inspiration. Envision a snapshot of reflection, where you interruption to recognize the headway you've made, the difficulties you've survived, and the strength that has carried you to this point.

•A Letter to Your Future Self
Consider writing a letter to your future self in which you envision the person you want to be and capture the essence of your journey. Share your fantasies, praise the triumphs you expect to accomplish, and offer thanks for the examples advanced en route. This letter turns into a period container of your desires and a wellspring of motivation on your proceeded with way.

May you revel in the victories of today, relish the excursion of tomorrow, and commend the dynamic woven artwork of your masterfully carried out life.

Conclusion.

Dear Friend, At this turning point in our journey together, it is time to begin the final chapter, one of self-awareness and empowerment. This is the decision, of a progression of sections, yet of an extraordinary endeavor toward a better, more joyful you.

• Reflecting on Your Journey.

1.The Embroidery of Moments.

Consider the intricate web of events that has woven your individual journey for a moment. Review the difficulties confronted, the triumphs celebrated, and the illustrations learned. You are the person you are right now because of every small or big step you've taken.

2. Development In the midst of Challenges:

Recognize the development that arose out of difficulties. Challenges are not barriers; they are open doors for flexibility, learning, and strength. Your perseverance and determination are clearly demonstrated by your capacity to overcome these obstacles.

3. Observe Your Wins:

Commend your successes, both of all shapes and sizes. The reliable decisions, the snapshots of self-restraint, and the examples where you focused on your prosperity — they all merit adulation. Your successes are the achievements that mark the way of your excursion.

4. Examples in Setbacks:

View misfortunes as examples as opposed to disappointments. Each diversion is an opportunity to reconsider, learn, and turn. It's through these misfortunes that you gain understanding, strengthen your purpose, and set up for considerably more noteworthy victories.

•Empowered Eating for a Healthier, Happier You.

1. A Careful Relationship with Food:

Engaged eating is tied in with encouraging a careful relationship with food. It's perceiving that each chomp is a chance to support your body and soul. Move toward dinners with expectation, relishing the flavors and embracing the sustenance they give.

2. The Force of Choice:

Your process has featured the force of decision — the ability to pick food sources that elevate, stimulate, and maintain. Each decision is a stage toward a better, more joyful you. Engaged eating is tied in with settling on decisions lined up with your prosperity while recognizing that equilibrium is vital.

3. Happy Development and Well-Being:

Past the plate, commend the delight of development and its significant effect on prosperity. Whether it's a dance, a walk around nature, or a heart-siphoning exercise, development is a festival of what your body can accomplish. Allow it to be a wellspring of delight as opposed to an errand.

• An Intelligent Second

Presently, we should take part in a snapshot of connection. Think about the accompanying inquiries:
- What is one test you defeated during your excursion that you are especially glad for?
- Consider a little success that gave monstrous pleasure. What was it, and how did your journey change as a result?
- How has your relationship with food developed? Are there explicit decisions or propensities that have changed to improve things?

Feel free to write down your thoughts, share them with a friend, or even draw a picture of them.

This collaboration is an individual designated spot — an affirmation of your development and a festival of the remarkable way you've voyaged.

As we finish up this intuitive note, recollect that your process is a continuous embroidered artwork, persistently formed by your decisions, encounters, and reflections. Every second, whether a crossroads or a delicate bend, adds extravagance to the story of your masterfully carried out life.

May your way be decorated with the shades of self-revelation, strengthening, and the steadfast conviction that a better, more joyful you is a developing magnum opus.

Wellness wishes
(Catherine.J.Norris)

Your Review Matters:

If you've had the pleasure of diving into [Dine Smart, Win Big], we invite you to share your thoughts. Your reviews contribute to the tapestry of experiences, helping others discover the transformative power within these pages. Join the conversation and let your voice be heard!